namaste

We hope you enjoy learning about Ayuryoga through this introductory booklet on the three doshas: vata, pitta, and kapha. By understanding the meaning of how each dosha's physiology, qualities, and association with the elements and senses brings forth their actions, you can tailor your practice to bring harmony and balance. We recommend receiving instruction from a certified Ayuryoga teacher or Yoga professional.

All Ayuryoga protocols have a pranayama component. You can start with pranayama and follow minimum recommendations. Meditation is important to relax the mind and nervous system so in the morning or evening try one of the recommended meditations. Then explore either the namaskar or asana recommendations. Practice on an empty stomach, preferably sometime between 6:00 to 9:00 AM and 5:00 to 8:00 PM. Meditation can happen anytime throughout the day. Blending this information will take practice and experience to find the perfect balance for you.

Think Prakruti

In essence, we are made up of all three doshas. However, we have unique proportions of each dosha and that makes us unique. Choose the practice recommendation that corresponds with your primary dosha. Or choose from both primary and secondary doshas and create a mixed practice.

Think Vikruti

When we challenge our natural constitutional balance with aggravating diet and lifestyle choices then we fall into a state of imbalance called vikruti. When we are in this state, it is important to pacify the dosha that is most prevalent in the imbalanced state while also choosing some of the practices that are part of your prakruti.

Think Seasonally

The shift and change in seasons can cause imbalance to our prakruti. While doing our best to maintain balance, we need to pacify the doshas using seasonal principles. Therefore, in the summer, follow the pitta program and in the fall, follow the vata program. Vata and kapha combine for winter practices, while spring is generally kapha management time. These principles vary depending on where you live and how each season expresses the elements and qualities associated with the dosha.

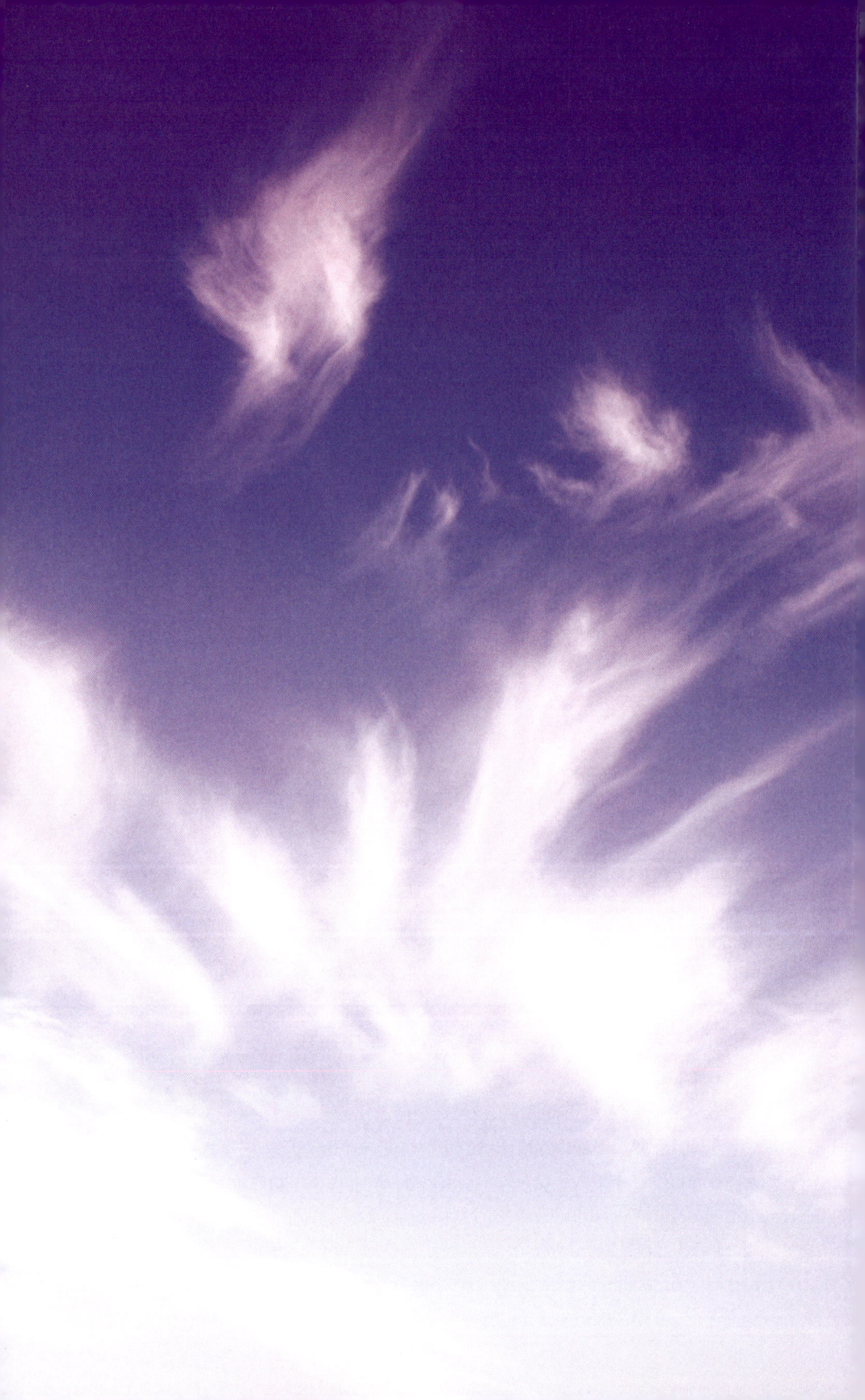

vata

THE ENERGY OF MOVEMENT
The principles of sensory stimuli and motor responses

SUB-DOSHAS

PRANA VAYU
head/brain
movement of
thoughts and senses
mentation

UDANA VAYU
diaphragm to throat
exhalation
speech
expression
memory function

SAMANA VAYU
small intestines
navel
digestive secretions

APANA VAYU
pelvic cavity
exhalation
elimination
downward movement

VYANA VAYU
heart
circulation

Vata dosha predominates in all bodily movement in the form of sensory stimuli and motor responses. A vata-dominant person is blessed with a quick and creative mind, flexibility, and creativity. Mentally, they usually grasp concepts quickly but then forget them just as quickly. Alert, restless, and very active, vata people walk, talk, and think fast, but are easily fatigued. They always take the initiative and are very lively in conversation, are quick to answer without thinking. Physically they have: a lean body, dry skin, curly/kinky hair, cold hands and feet, variable digestion tending towards bloating, discomfort and constipation. Their sleep is light and most of their lifestyle routines are irregular.

When unbalanced, vata types may become fearful, nervous, and anxious. They are not good planners and consequently may suffer economic hardship. They tend to have less willpower, confidence, boldness, and tolerance than other types and often feel unstable and ungrounded. Prone to worry, they often have anxiety, stress, and, when under stress, they are easily fatigued and confused about that they did wrong. They can become impulsive, compulsive, and erratic.

ELEMENTS
Space, Air

GUNAS
cold, dry, light, mobile,
subtle, clear, rough

ORGANS AND MAIN SITES
colon and pelvic cavity, legs,
thighs, ears, skin, bones

**EMOTIONS AND
NATURAL ABILITIES**
fear, insecurity, anxiety, prone to
excitability, creativity, adaptability,
and changeability

IMBALANCES
insomnia, lack of focus, stress/
anxiety, mental worries, transient
hypertension, gas, constipation,
sciatica, overactive, underweight,
twitches, aching or cracking joints

TIME
dawn and dusk
2:00 to 6:00 AM and PM
4 hours after a meal

SEASON
fall, early winter

COLORS
purple, blue, black, brown

BALANCING COLORS
warming colors
orange, yellow, red

SPICES
cinnamon, cardamom, clove,
mustard, asafetida, ginger

Vata provides the essential motion and direction for all bodily processes to occur. Vata is most prominent in the fall and early winter seasons, so these are the most important times to be careful of diet and lifestyle schedule and routine. Establishing a consistent routine is a key consideration for balancing vata dosha.

Vata dosha resides in the colon, as well as the brain, ears, bones, joints, skin, and thighs. Vata people are susceptible to diseases involving the air principle, such as emphysema, pneumonia, and arthritis. Other common vata disorders include flatulence, tics, twitches, aching joints, ringing in the ear, dry skin and hair, nerve disorders, constipation, and mental confusion. Vata dosha tends to increase with age as is indicated by drying and wrinkling of the skin and erosion of the body.

Since the attributes of vata dosha are dry, light, cold, rough, subtle, mobile, and clear, any of these qualities in excess can cause imbalance. Frantic travel, especially by plane, loud noises, continual stimulation, drugs, sugar, caffeine, and alcohol all derange vata, as do exposure to cold and cold foods. Like the wind, vata types have a hard time getting and staying grounded. Routine is difficult but essential if vata dosha is to be balanced and controlled. It best for vata types to go to bed early, as they need more rest than other types. In general, people with excessive vata respond most rapidly to warm, moist, slightly oily, heavy foods. Steam baths, humidifiers, and moisture in general are also helpful. Daily abhyanga (oil massage) before bath or shower is also recommended with sesame or almond oil. Even abhyanga before yoga practice with a warm shower can be highly beneficial for vata types.

General guidelines for balancing vata
- Keep warm and avoid drafts
- Stay calm and focused and avoid multi-tasking
- Rest and avoid expending energy all at once
- Avoid cold, frozen, and raw foods
- Eat warm foods and spices
- Maintain a regular routine

Ayuryoga for Vata

To balance the natural attributes of vata, emphasize the opposite qualities and elements: Earth, Water, and Fire offer stable, slow, heavy, and warm qualities along with other gunas such as the oily, liquid, smooth, gross and sticky qualities. When these principles are applied within asana, there is an emphasis on stabilizing and grounding the foundation of the pose, giving attention to muscular energy and alignment to invite the stable, heavy and slow qualities to the practice. Oily, liquid, and smooth qualities can be incorporated into the practice by focusing on smooth movements, moving with the breath, and avoiding movements that are quick, jerky, or frenetic.

It is best for vata types to practice in a warm, draft-free room and move slowly, focusing on a steady movement with mindfulness of maintaining an even breath. Pacing the practice is important, as vata people usually like to expend energy all at once, moving quickly, and then tire more easily. Therefore, they need to learn to conserve energy with slower, mindful movements instead of quickly expending it.

Vata types can tend toward hypermobile joints and therefore can seem quite flexible in most asanas; however, this can quickly lead to injury. Those with light and overly limber joints should focus on strength and stability rather than flexibility.

PRANAYAMA FOR VATA

Agni Sara

Anuloma Viloma *best*

Bhramari

Kapalabhati

Nadi Shodhana

Utgeet

Utjayi

PRANAYAMA

Vata people generally exhale easier than they inhale. They must learn to increase the capacity of their inhalation.

MEDITATION

Meditation is very important for vata types because this is the best way to calm their hyperactive mind, which then leads to a hyperactive lifestyle. Structured meditation is best such as So'hum or Jappa Mala. In addition, they should schedule daily mediation at the same time of the day to support overall routine and good habits.

ASANA

Those with vata dosha predominant should focus on asanas that activate the pelvis, hip and thigh areas as these are the major sites for vata.

Standing poses stabilize and ground; provide strength and stability. Focus on apana vayu, grounding and anchoring. Balancing asana will help focus the mind and connect to the earth principle.

Forward bends release tension from the lower back (these stretch the lower back), heat the internal organs, and soothe the nervous system. They can balance apana and prana vayu.

Backbends on the belly are best to help stabilize any sacral instabiity or hypermobility. They also help warm the lower back and bring heat to the spine through extension. They can balance vyana, samana and udana vayu.

Inversions can support vata's weak digestive and ciculatory system. However due to their smaller, thinner bone tissue structure, vata types should not hold these asanas for very long. These can balance all vayus (samana and vyana can be a focus).

Examples of Vata Asanas See also Surya Namaskar on page 20

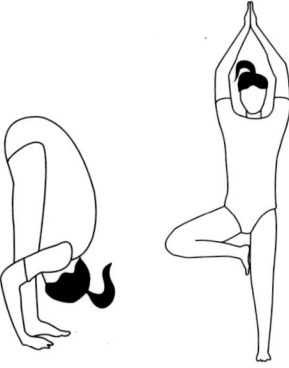
Uttanasana
standing forward bend

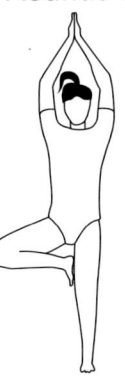
Vrksasana
tree pose

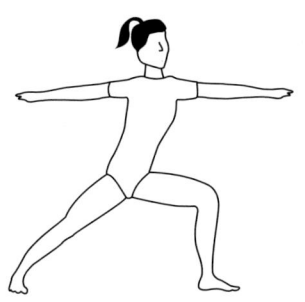
Virabhadrasana II
warrior pose II

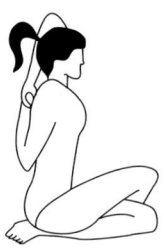
Gomukhasana
cow face pose

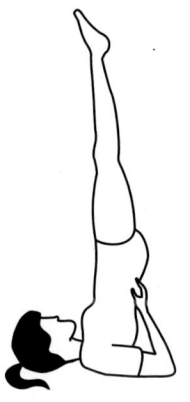
Salamba Sarvangasana
shoulderstand

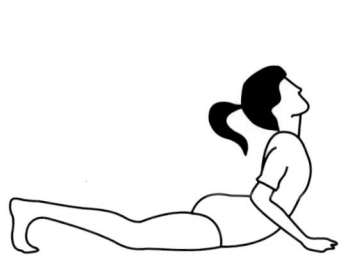
Bhujangasana
cobra pose

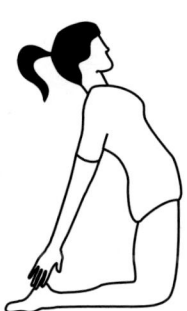
Ustrasana
camel pose

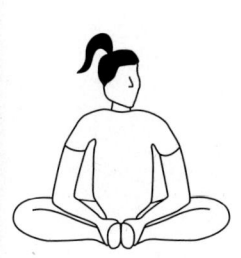
Baddha Konasana
bound angle pose

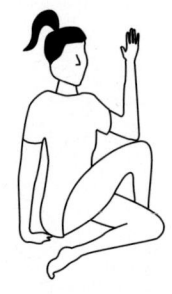
Ardha Matsyendrasana
half spinal twist

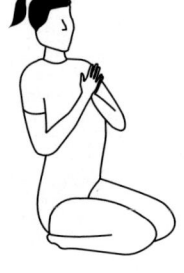
Vajrasana
thunderbolt pose

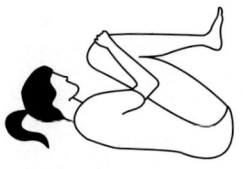
Pawanmuktasana
wind release pose

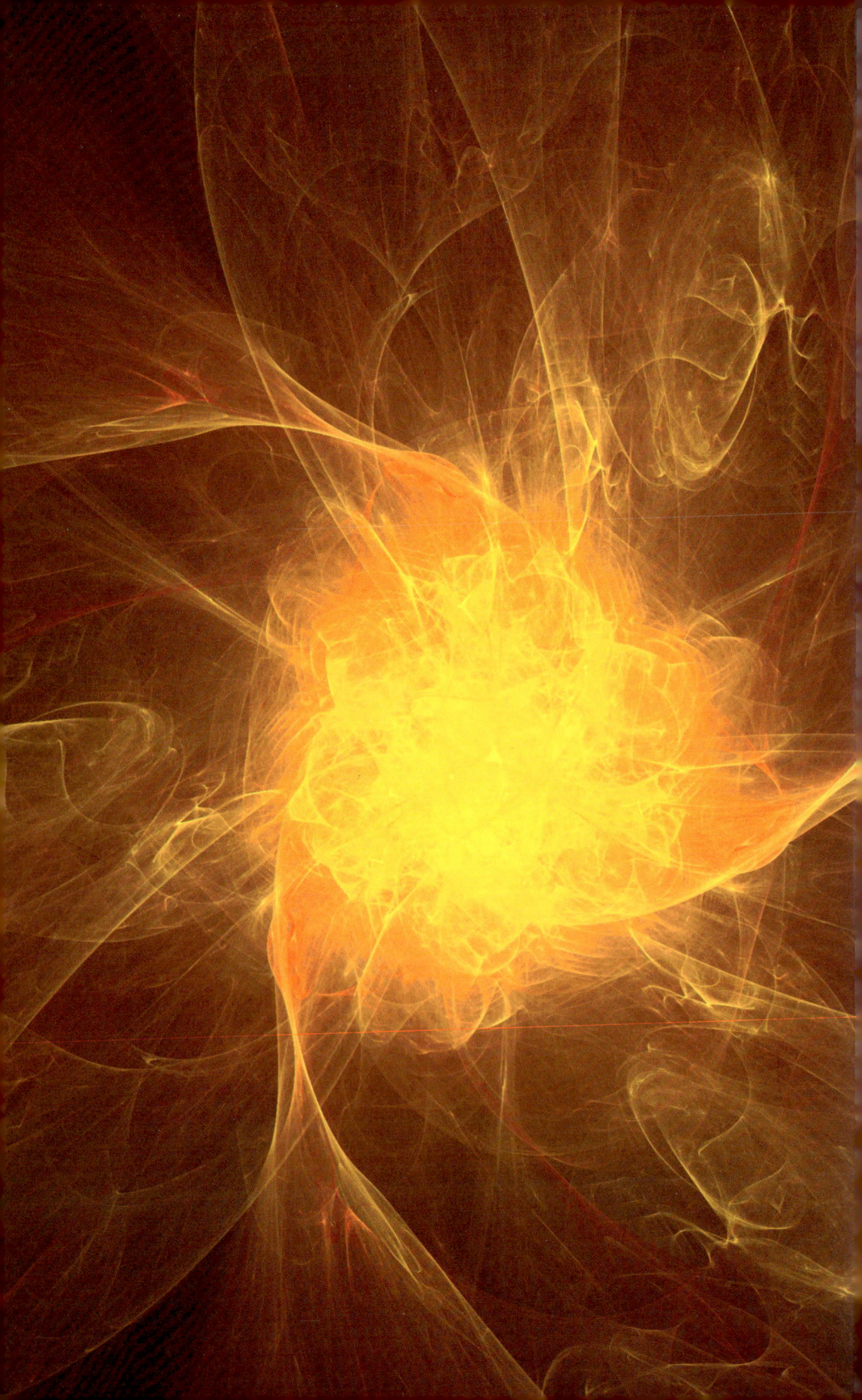

pitta

THE ENERGY OF TRANSFORMATION
The fire principle of metabolic activity and intellectual understanding

SUB-DOSHAS

SADHAKA PITTA
brain
thinking
emotions
conscious action

ALOCHAKA PITTA
optical perception

RANJAKA PITTA
liver
spleen
stomach/root of rakta
blood

PACHAKA PITTA
GI tract
digestion
absorption
assimilation

BHRAJAKA PITTA
metabolic processes
within the skin
melatonin

Pitta people embody the qualities of Fire and Water. Fire is hot, penetrating, sharp, and agitating while Water provides the oily quality. Therefore, pitta people have warm bodies, oily skin, penetrating ideas, and sharp intelligence. Pitta is responsible for body temperature, color complexion, knowledge, and understanding. These same qualities can also yield into agitation and a short temper. The pitta body type is one of medium height and build with ruddy or coppery skin. Their skin is warm and sensitive and may have many moles and freckles. Their hair tends to be straight, thin, and shiny and they often experience premature graying or hair loss (receding hairline). Pitta types have a bright, brilliant intellectual look with sharp, sensitive eyes. Their eyes are of medium size and can tend toward irritation. The nose is sharp and the tip tends to be reddish. They can easily perspire, have warm hands and feet, tend towards red rashes, multiple acne spots, and skin sensitivity to sunlight. Pitta people have a lower tolerance for sunlight, heat, or hard physical work.

Pitta individuals have a strong metabolism, good digestion, and good appetite, but can tend

ELEMENTS
Fire, Water

GUNAS
hot, sharp, penetrating, light, oily, liquid, spreading

ORGANS AND MAIN SITES
small intestine, navel, liver, gallbladder, spleen, sweat and blood

EMOTIONS AND NATURAL ABILITIES
ambition, irritability, jealousy, anger, sharp intellect, aggressiveness, thirst for knowledge, leadership, good concentration

IMBALANCES
diarrhea, ulcers, acid indigestion, skin conditions, migraine headache, recurrent fevers

TIME
mid-day and midnight
10:00 to 2:00 AM and PM
2 hours after a meal

SEASON
summer

COLORS
red, yellow, and orange

BALANCING COLORS
cooling colors
white, blue, green

SPICES
cumin, coriander, fennel, mint

toward acid indigestion. They enjoy consuming plenty of food and liquids. They usually love hot spices and cold drinks; however, they need sweet, bitter, and astringent tastes to bring balance. They produce large quantities of urine and feces, which tend to be yellowish, oily, soft, and plentiful.

Mentally, pitta types are alert and intelligent and have good comprehension. They always carry a book in their hand, as they like to fuel the mind with reading, solving puzzles and doing calculations. However, they are easily agitated, competitive, and aggressive and, when out of balance, tend toward hatred, anger, and jealousy. In the external world, pitta people like to be leaders and planners and seek material prosperity, exhibiting their wealth and possessions.

Since the attributes of pitta are oily, hot, light, mobile, and liquid, an excess of any of these qualities can cause aggravation that shows up as fevers and inflammatory conditions, for example. Common symptoms include skin rashes, rosacea, ulcerations, fever, inflammation, or irritations such as conjunctivitis, colitis, or gastritis. Summer is pitta season; therefore, sunburn, poison ivy, heat exhaustion, and irritability are more common at this time. Diet and lifestyle should focus on cooling foods and environment. They should eat foods that are sweet, bitter, and astringent, and do activities that rest the body and mind. Abhyanga with coconut or sunflower oil is best for pitta skin.

General guidelines for balancing pitta
- Avoid excessive heat
- Avoid excessive oil
- Avoid excessive steam
- Limit salt intake
- Eat cooling, non-spicy foods
- Exercise during the cooler part of the day

Ayuryoga for Pitta

In Ayurveda, we apply opposite attributes, or guna(s), to alleviate doshic imbalances. Since pitta is hot, sharp, light, spreading, and penetrating, it can be balanced by the cool, dry, dull, soft, and dark qualities.

It is important to target the areas where pitta is more prevalent in the body such as the navel or solar plexus area as well the liver and small intestine, to release tension and heat from these organs. Asanas that stretch these areas will release heat and stagnation along with lowering excess heat from the head. Pitta individuals tend to accumulate too much heat in the head from excessive thinking and processing; the vata sub-dosha apana vayu will help move excess energy down. For a pitta type, staying cool is important so practicing in a well-ventilated room, that is not too bright, can help them stay cool and calm.

PRANAYAMA

Pitta people generally exhale faster than they inhale; therefore, they need to increase the volume of their exhalation to cool the body.

Sheetkari is similar in its effects to sheetali. For this pranayama, first flatten the tongue, then catch it between the teeth while stretching the mouth (like smiling) and inhaling through the teeth. This will cool the body and mind instantaneously. It is pitta-pacifying and neutral to vata and kapha.

PRANAYAMA FOR PITTA

Agni Sara

Chandra Bedhana

Kapalabhati

Sheetali *best*

Sheetkari *best*

MEDITATION

Pitta people should do a more passive form of meditation like Empty Bowl. They will also benefit from unstructured meditation practices. You can find instructions for Empty Bowl meditation on our website Ayurveda.com/online_resource.

ASANA

Asanas should be practiced with attention to the navel and solar plexus areas. Backward bending helps release excess heat from the sites where pitta tends to accumulate. Lateral flexion and twists can also help detoxify excess pitta. Forward bends tend to heat the internal organs and should be avoided or not held for a long period of time, especially standing forward bends.

Standing poses can increase heat since it involves using major muscles. Standing asana that stretch the lower torso and side body will release excess pitta.

Back bends in general will pacify pitta dosha from the body. Those that are on the belly can activate important marma points that also benefit pitta.

Twisting is harmonizing and balancing as it stretches and compresses major organs within the solar plexus.

Inversions should be done with great caution as inversions that place the head perpendicular to the floor like Sirsasana (headstand) will bring heat and blood to the head and often elevate pitta dosha. However, other inversions like Sarvangasana (shoulder stand) can be beneficial to cool excess heat in the nervous system.

Examples of Pitta Asanas See also Chandra Namaskar on page 22

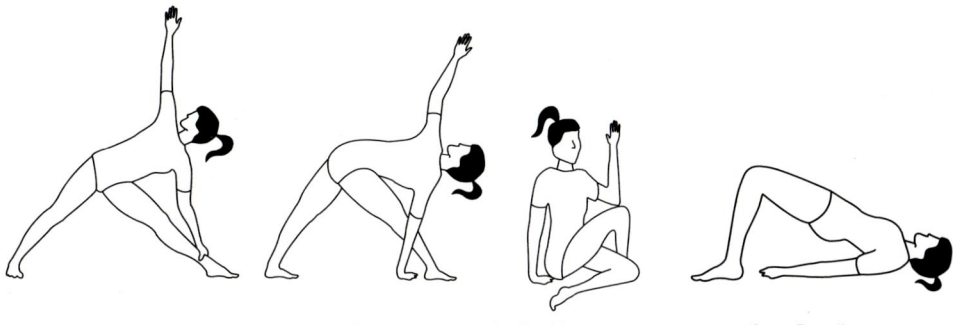

Utthita Trikonasana
triangle pose

Parivrrta Trikonasana
revolved triangle pose

Ardha Matsyendrasana
half spinal twist

Setu Bandhasana
bridge pose

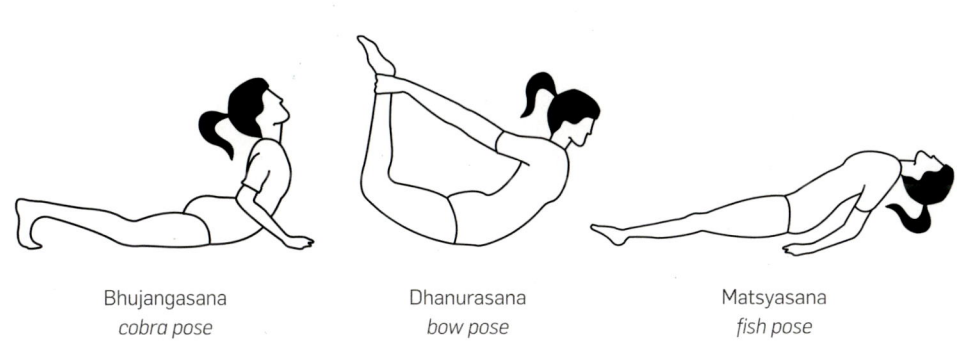

Bhujangasana
cobra pose

Dhanurasana
bow pose

Matsyasana
fish pose

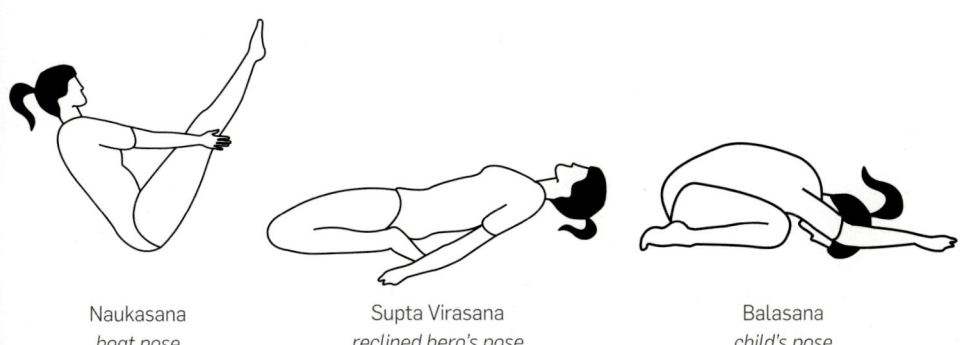

Naukasana
boat pose

Supta Virasana
reclined hero's pose

Balasana
child's pose

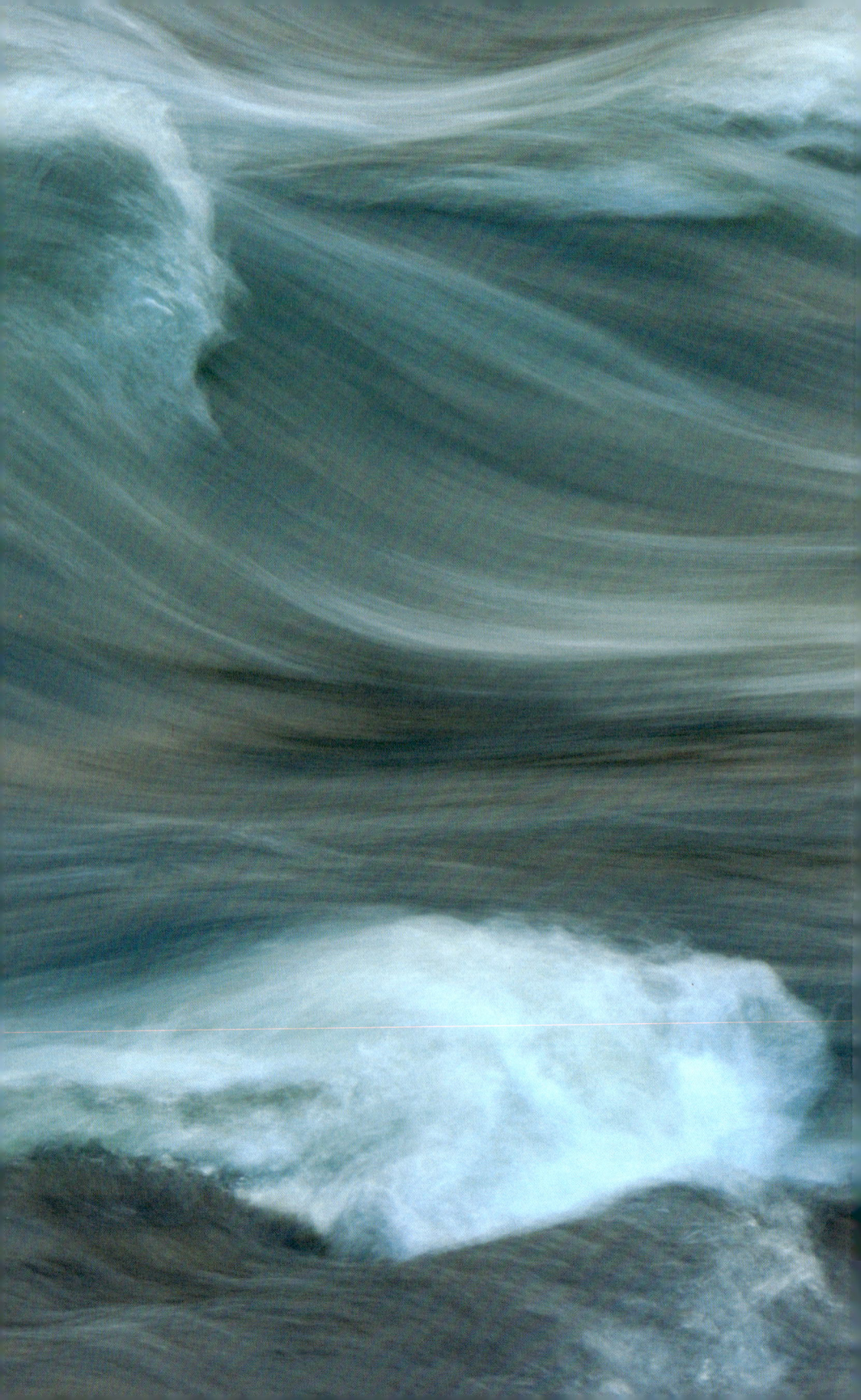

kapha

THE ENERGY OF LUBRICATION
The earth principle of building block material

SUB-DOSHAS

KLEDAKA KAPHA
stomach
GI track

AVALAMBAKA KAPHA
lungs
pleural cavity
heart
respiratory tract
thoracic spine

BODHAKA KAPHA
oral cavity

TARPAKA KAPHA
brain
myelin sheath
cerebral spinal fluid

SHLESHAKA KAPHA
general lubrication
especially in the joints

Kapha individuals tend to be calm, tolerant, and forgiving and are blessed with strength, stamina, and endurance. In balance, they are passive, stable and grounded. People with a kapha-dominant constitution have a large, physically strong body frame with well-developed muscles, cold, clammy, oily, porcelain white skin, and big, beautiful blue eyes with long, thick eyelashes and eyebrows.

Kapha people tend to gain weight easily due to a constitutionally slow metabolism and because they generally do not like to exercise. They have thick skin. They evacuate feces slowly and it tends to be soft, pale, and oily. Perspiration is moderate. Sleep is deep and prolonged.

Their mental capacity can seem sluggish as they are slow to comprehend, but their long term memory is excellent and, once they learn something, they never forget it. They are very forgiving, compassionate, and loving. However, when kapha dosha is out of balance, they can experience greed, attachment, possessiveness, and depression.

Kapha types are usually attracted to sweet, salty, and oily foods, but their bodies need bitter, astringent, and pungent tastes. They tend to have diseases connected to the Earth and Water

ELEMENTS
Water, Earth

GUNAS
heavy, slow/dull, cold, oily, liquid, slimy/smooth, dense, soft, static, sticky, cloudy, hard, and gross

ORGANS AND MAIN SITES
lungs, stomach, sinuses, lymphatics, adipose tissue

EMOTIONS AND NATURAL ABILITIES
attachment, greed, comforting, compassion, loving, forgiving, stable, strong

IMBALANCES
cold, congestion, and cough, edema, weight gain, depression, slow metabolism, feelings of heaviness and lethargy, excessive sleep

TIME
early morning and evening
6:00 to 10:00 AM and PM
soon after a meal

SEASON
late winter, spring

COLORS
white, grey, light blue

BALANCING COLORS
red, orange, blue/purple, like the sky

SPICES
mustard, cayenne pepper, turmeric, trikatu (ginger, black pepper, piper longum)

elements such as the flu, excess mucous or sinus congestion, and edema. Sluggishness, excess weight, diabetes, water retention, and congestive headache are also common. Late winter and spring is the time of greatest kapha accumulation, so following a kapha-balancing diet and lifestyle are most important during that time. Self-massage (abhyanga) with corn, mustard, or sesame oil is best. Physical activity will help release stagnation, invigorating the body and mind to feel light and bright.

General guidelines for balancing kapha

- Get plenty of exercise
- Avoid heavy foods such as beef, cheese, or yogurt
- Keep active
- Avoid dairy
- Avoid iced food or drinks
- Vary your routine
- Avoid fatty, oily or fried foods
- Eat light, dry food
- No daytime naps

Ayuryoga for Kapha

The elements of Earth and Water predominate in the kapha type body and mind and manifest as the following qualities: heavy, slow/dull, cool, oily, liquid, slimy/smooth, dense, soft, static, sticky/cloudy, and gross. To counter these attributes, a yoga practice should be light and expansive with a rhythmic pace and progressively challenging asanas. Kapha constitution is balanced by a vigorous, challenging asana practice that builds heat and induces sweating. The soft, gross, and sticky/cloudy qualities can manifest in the body as excess adipose tissue and in the mind as a lack of motivation and clarity. Motivation to commit to a regular yoga practice can be challenging for kapha types, as they generally do not like to exercise. Once they begin to experience the benefits of movement, they will become attached to this new sense of well-being and will easily sustain a regular, daily practice. Of all the doshas, kapha is endowed with great strength and stamina so they can sustain a longer and more challenging yoga practice.

When there is excess kapha, one will feel heavy and stagnant and not want to move in a vigorous way. Since kapha can accumulate in the lymphatic system and adipose tissue, steady movement will move and disperse stagnant fluids in the body. Therefore, it is recommended to begin moving slowly to move stagnation and denseness then progress to a stronger, more challenging practice once they feel lighter.

PRANAYAMA

The main site of kapha is the chest area and accumulation here can lead to congestion, heavy breathing, and mouth breathing. Pranayama is important to help release this excess buildup and to lighten the body and mind, so they can more easily do asana.

MEDITATION

Kapha types like to sit so meditation can be easy for them. However, dullness and heaviness in the mind can make meditation very dull. Therefore, structured meditation such as Trataka (ghee lamp gazing) and moving/walking meditations can be very good for kapha dosha.

PRANAYAMA FOR KAPHA

Agni Sara

Bhastrika *best*

Bhramari

Kapalabhati

ASANA

Vigorous and challenging asanas are suggested; therefore, they can hold or stay in asana for a longer period of time than other dosha types. It is important to stretch and open the torso and chest areas. Also, doing asanas that increase heart rate may help reduce excess weight.

Standing poses are kapha-reducing, especially those in which the arms are raised above the shoulders. It is good to lift the energy up from the pelvic floor and open the chest, the seat of kapha dosha.

Back bends are kapha-reducing because of the strong opening they bring to the chest and lungs, the main site of kapha. More strenuous backbends, such as Urdhva Dhanurasana (upward bow or wheel) are best. Most backbends also stimulate the thyroid gland, which tends to be sluggish, improving its function.

Forward bends will bring heat to the chest, which can help offset the cold, damp qualities that create excess kapha. Standing forward bends are more active than seated ones.

Inversions can be beneficial for kapha types, as it stimulates lymphatic circulation and can bring a feeling of lightness to the body. Be cautious if there is excess weight on the body because this can create strain on the cervical spine.

Examples of Kapha Asanas See also Surya Namaskar on page 20

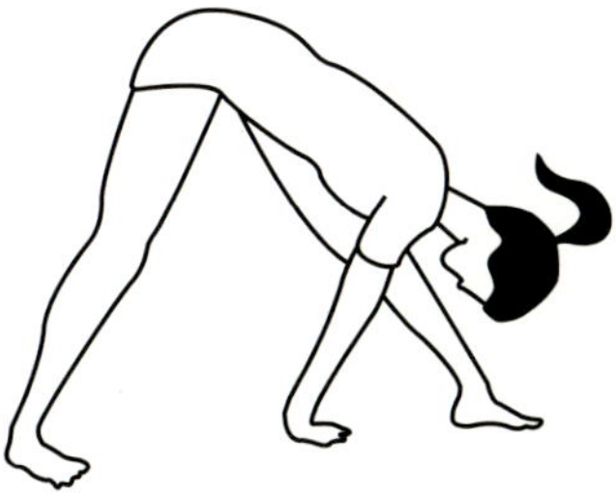

Parsvottanasana
pyramid pose

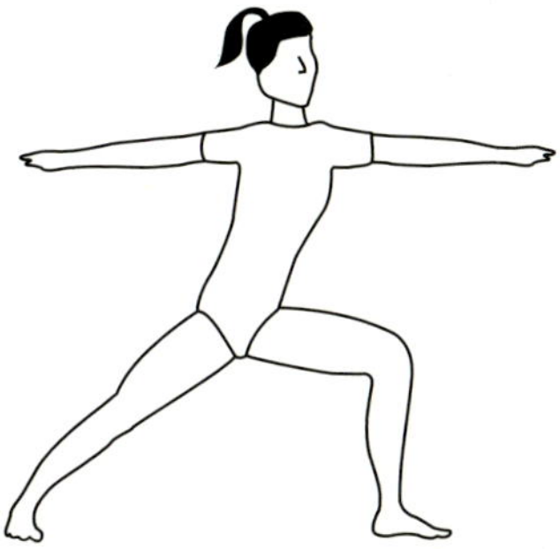

Virabhadrasana II
warrior pose II

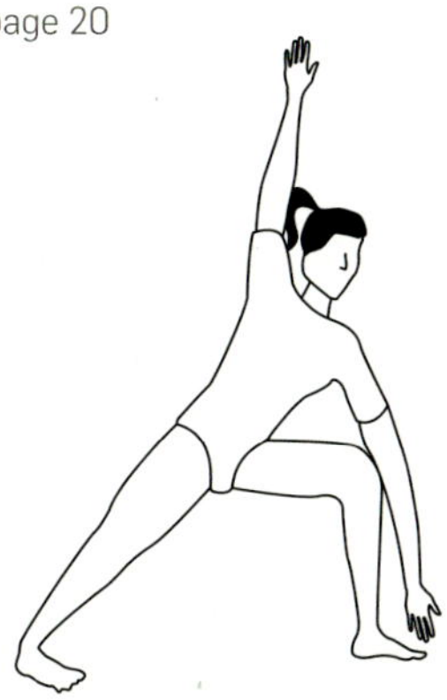

Utthita Parsvakonasana
extended side angle pose

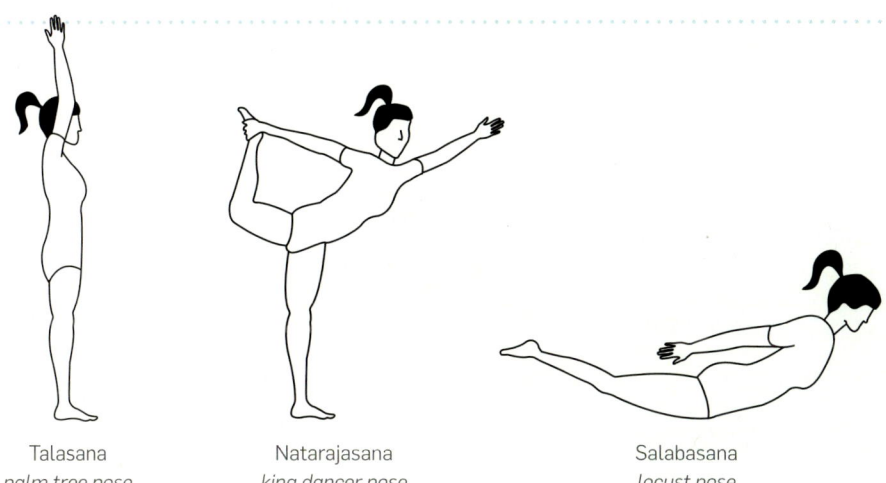

Talasana
palm tree pose

Natarajasana
king dancer pose

Salabasana
locust pose

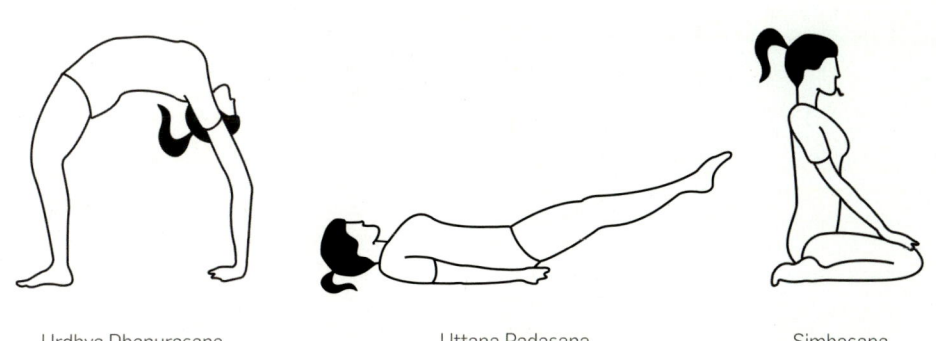

Urdhva Dhanurasana
wheel pose

Uttana Padasana
raised legs pose

Simhasana
lion pose

Surya Namaskar

Vata types practice slow and steady with a focus on the pelvis, hip and thigh areas

Kapha types practice vigorously being mindful to stretch and open the torso and chest areas

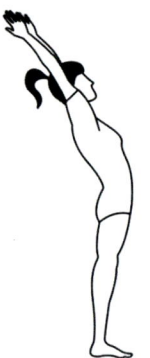

Parvatasana
inhale

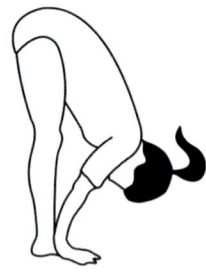

Hasta Padasana
exhale

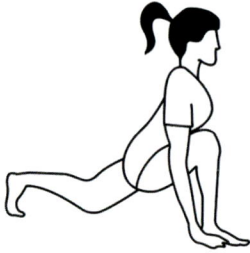

Eka Pada Prasarasana
inhale

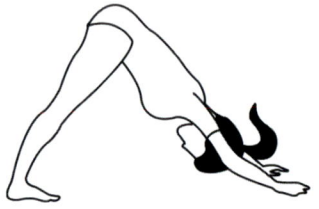

Bhudharasana
exhale

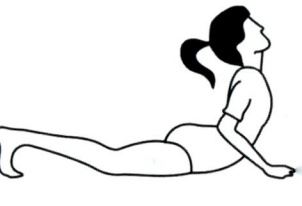

Bhujangasana
inhale

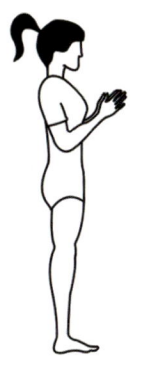

START ▶
Dakshasana

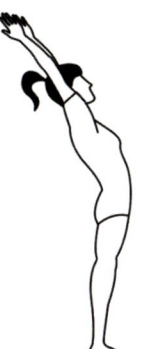

Parvatasana
inhale

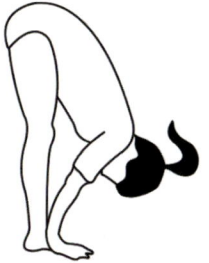

Hasta Padasana
exhale

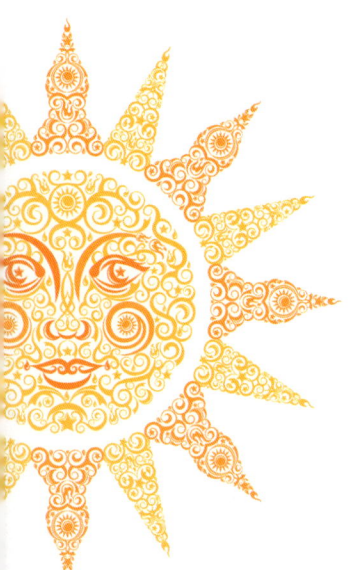

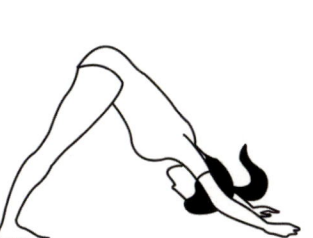

Eka Pada Prasarasana
inhale

Bhudharasana
exhale

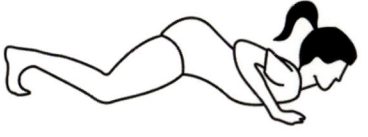

Asthanga Pranipatasana

Chandra Namaskar

Pitta types practice with attention to the navel and solar plexus areas

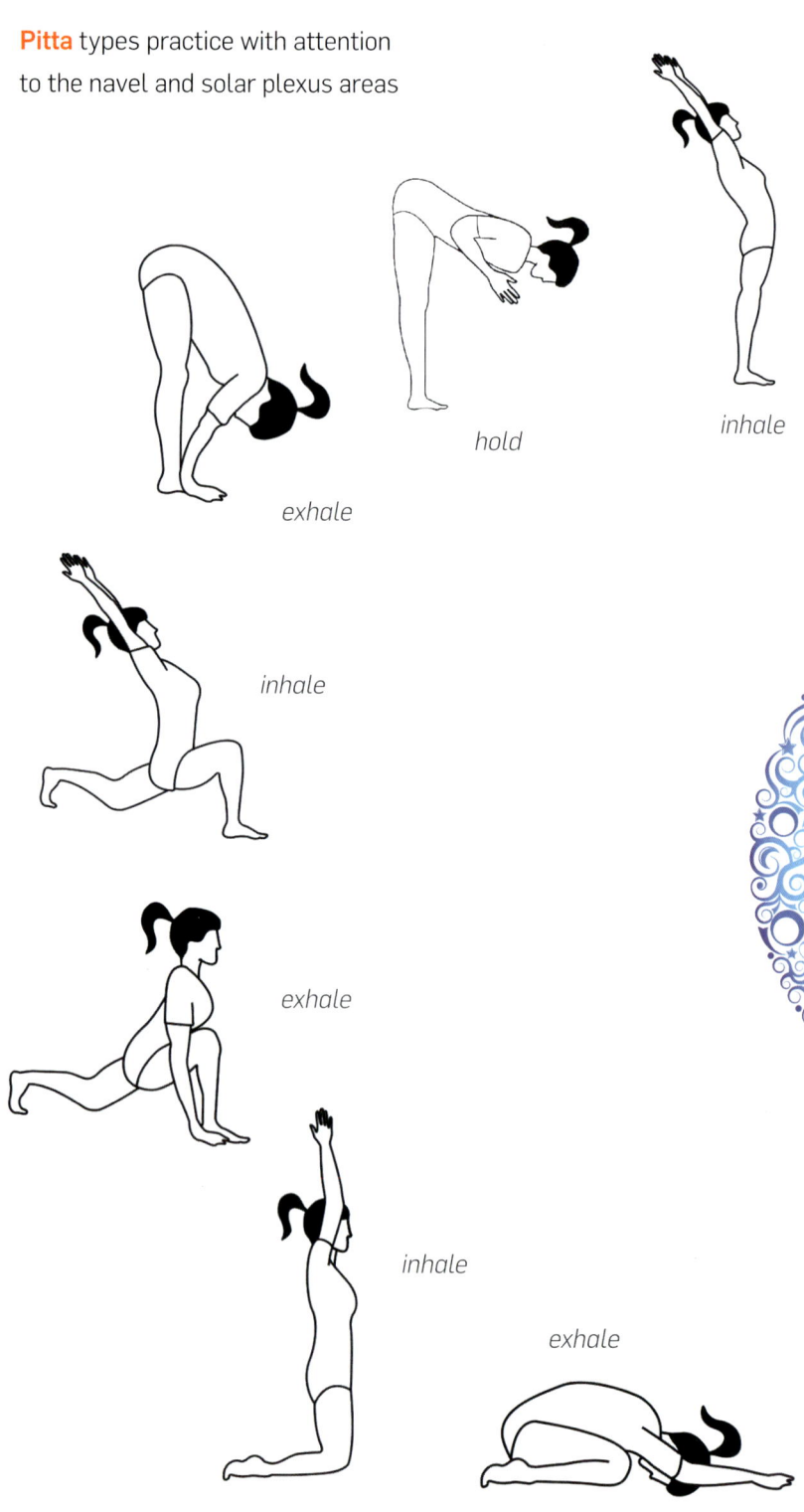

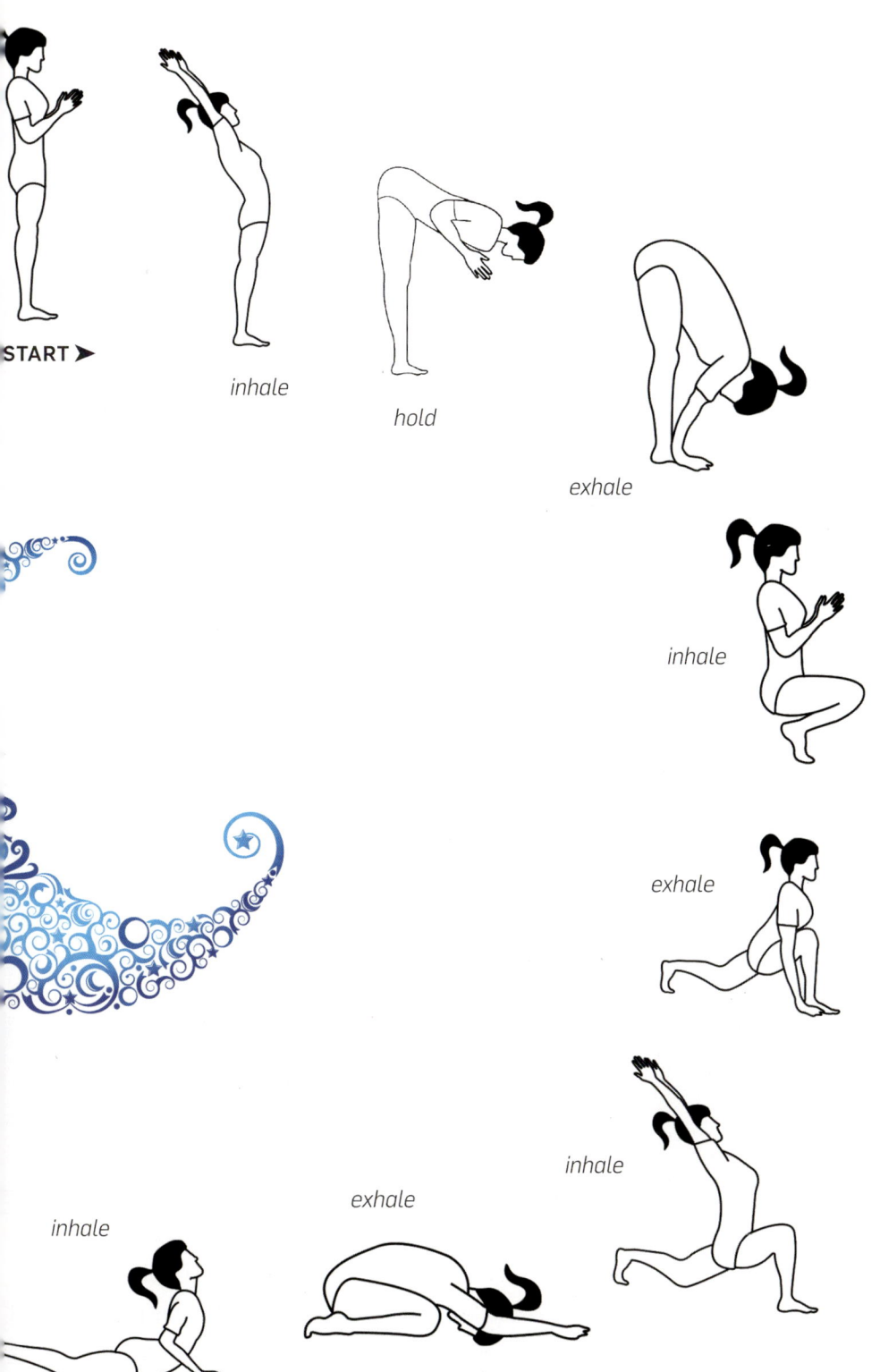

about the authors

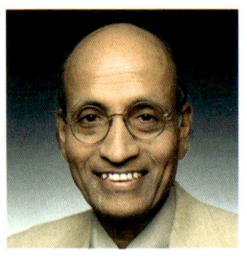

Vasant Lad, BMA&S, MASc, Ayurvedic Physician

Vasant Lad brings a wealth of classroom and practical experience to the United States. A native of India, he served for three years as Medical Director of the Ayurveda Hospital in Pune, India. He was Professor of Clinical Medicine at the Pune University College of Ayurvedic Medicine for 15 years. He holds a Bachelor's of Ayurvedic Medicine and Surgery (BAM&S) degree from the University of Pune and a Master's of Ayurvedic Science (MASc) degree from Tilak Ayurved Mahavidyalaya. Vasant Lad's academic and practical training include the study of Allopathy (Western medicine) and surgery as well as traditional Ayurveda.

Beginning in 1979, he has traveled throughout the United States sharing his knowledge of Ayurveda. In 1984 he came to Albuquerque as Director, principal instructor and founder of the Ayurvedic Institute. Vasant Lad is the author of numerous books and respected throughout the world for his knowledge of Ayurveda. Vasant Lad is the author of 11 books on Ayurveda as well as hundreds of articles and other writings. With over 500,000 copies of his books in print in the US, his work has been translated into more than 20 languages.

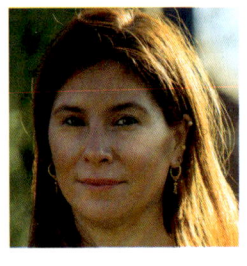

Maria E Garré, MEd, E-RYT-500

Head of the Ayuryoga Department, Maria teaches ASP 2 Ayuryoga, YTT, and online Ayuryoga. Maria is dedicated to a life-long study, practice, and teaching of both Yoga and Ayurveda; continuing over 20 years of study in Medical and Biological Sciences, Philosophy, Ayurveda and Yoga.

Blending the knowledge she has gathered from her studies and yearly pilgrimages to India, Maria leads dynamic and liberating classes that embody the alchemy of all these disciplines. Along with teaching at the Institute, Maria travels internationally leading retreats, workshops, and teacher training programs throughout the world.